Table of Contents

Strategies for Outdoor Activities with Allergies

1. Introduction to Outdoor Allergies

The incidence of allergic rhinitis has also been steadily increasing across the USA, and its presence can exacerbate asthma symptoms, leading people to believe they have both conditions. Allergic rhinitis can occur in four forms, classified primarily according to the duration of signs and symptoms (intermittent versus persistent) and severity (mild versus moderate-to-severe). Recent summer data for the 2017 Spring Allergy Capital shows pollen counts increasing throughout the season and impacting college athletes who suffer from allergy-induced asthma. Aerobic exercise increases the rate and depth of breathing, exposing athletes with allergic rhinitis to higher levels of allergens. Athletes coping with allergy-induced asthma are prone to more frequent asthma attacks if their allergic rhinitis is not well managed.

The term "outdoor allergies" refers to allergic reactions to substances commonly found in the great outdoors. Common triggers associated with outdoor allergies include pollen particles released by grasses, trees, and flowers, as well as airborne mold spores and stinging insects. Even an allergen-free outdoor activity can still cause discomfort, as physical exertion can cause people to breathe through their mouths, bypassing their bodies' first line of defense against outdoor allergens—the nasal passages. Allergic reactions to latex and insect venom can be especially problematic for outdoor sport enthusiasts as they may lead to itching, hives, swelling, and possibly severe anaphylactic shock.

1.1. Understanding Common Outdoor Allergens

In the active summer and spring months, insect allergies can quickly turn outdoor fun into a medical emergency. Exposure to insect venom can be dangerous for those who have allergies or who have been stung frequently by stinging insects. An "immediate" allergic reaction can happen if you've ever been stung by an insect—including a mild one that warrants a home treatment if stung, such as a mosquito—as well as those that present more severe risks. Online (open) allergy testing is not recommended for anyone. If you have positive results from an online allergy test, your veterinarian will discuss what testing is recommended.

Out of all outdoor allergens, pollen is the most notorious. Plants produce a lot of pollen, which is carried by the wind to fertilize other plants. Individual plant populations release their pollen at different times when you'll notice allergic symptoms if you're allergic to some pollens. Since populations differ from region to region, your pollen seasons might change if you travel somewhere. Mold is another allergen that occurs outside. Mold is a fungus that grows in damp locations from relatively allergen-free to spaces for water-related activities. Mold can cause symptoms all year long in certain locations. However, their durability and tendency to produce spores make them the most frequent cause of fall allergies.

The great outdoors provides a sense of adventure and peace that's hard to find indoors. Outdoor activities do have their own unique risks, however; outdoor allergens can spell trouble for some individuals. Allergens are substances that can cause allergic reactions. Your body releases a compound called histamine if your immune system misidentifies an allergen as a harmful substance.

2. Preparation Before Heading Out

These individuals, who are referred to as atopic, should consult an allergist who has the specialized training required to diagnose and develop a custom management strategy or care plan for their precise problem. After an entire history and physical examination, the allergist may recommend testing the patient for allergies. In the office, the care provider can examine the body's reaction to allergens before recommending an allergy shot (immunotherapy). In case experience suggests that the patient is at risk of anaphylaxis, the doctor may offer an epinephrine auto-injector prescription. Afterwards, they should teach individuals who ought to take the medicine how to do so and when one can avoid the drug as well.

Before heading out, those with allergy concerns might consider several strategies to prevent their next adventure from casually unfolding into a medical emergency. Early preparation is particularly necessary as outdoor activities such as hikes and even unexpected walks can subject individuals to unexpected outdoor triggers. Any individual that has not fully investigated his or her allergies, particularly those whose immune system is overly sensitive to specific allergens, is at the greatest risk of a dangerous allergic reaction.

2.1. Consulting with an Allergist

Consulting with an allergist before engaging in outdoor activities is the most proactive approach to mitigating the occurrence of allergic symptoms. The allergist will assess a person's outdoor environment for known allergens so as to provide tailored, individual precautions. They will provide information about common airborne allergen triggers that can be seen in the local climate/environment and the recommended precautions to avoid allergic triggers, as well as the ideal time of year to visit a selected destination. The physical examination will be tailored to help manage the different types of allergies likely to occur in people who love outdoor activities so as to proactively manage the challenges posed by it.

It is wise to consult with an allergist before venturing out for outdoor activities. Communication with the allergist can be facilitated with a few steps such as discussing the duration of the trip, the medications and gear that they are ready to carry, any other health concerns, and mentioning a brief history of allergies that they have experienced or any physical anomalies. Severe allergies must be treated with caution and activities may need to be postponed or avoided if the risk is unduly high. Subsequently, a personalized list of contingencies will be offered that will range from first-aid at the campsite to medications and diagnostics should the need arise. Medication protocols, from the onset of allergies to treatment and cure, will be discussed in the following sections to different degrees, depending on the allergen.

3. Essential Gear and Supplies

Accessory options—some gear possibilities, in addition to treated or special clothing, include accessories that fit between the bumpers of a vehicle and help keep insects out of front- and back-of-vehicle sleeping accommodations.

Clothing can be treated with microencapsulated permethrin that slowly disperses to the surface of the garment, and is supposed to be an effective deterrent for insects coming into contact with the clothing. There is some evidence that permethrin may also help repel ticks.

Allergy-friendly Clothing and Gear Protective clothing reduces opportunities for allergens to make contact with the skin, in turn reducing allergic reactions. Clothing features: - Light, loose-weave fabric to allow some air exchange. - Elastic cuffs and elastic drawstrings to keep the clothing close to the skin and prevent allergens from getting inside. - Hoods and ventilating systems to allow some air exchange while minimizing allergens from entering the protective gear.

In addition to using repellents and taking medications, 50% of the practitioners included in a 2019 survey engaged in outdoor activities and made lifestyle choices to minimize insect exposure. Those choices included wearing protective clothing (45%) and avoiding known problem areas (44%). If you deal with outdoor allergies and insect sensitivities, protective clothing and gear can be a great resource. Here's an overview of what's available for those spending time outside.

3.1. Allergy-Friendly Clothing and Accessories

The American College of Allergy, Asthma, and Immunology (ACAAI) says that while the outdoors are rife with allergens, the body can be kept safe through protective gear and specific medications. Allergy-friendly clothing is available, offering a barrier to pests and pollens. Allergy clothing tends to be made of tightly woven materials or closed-knitting structures, and protective patches are added to prevent outbreaks or more serious allergic reactions. Along with allergy clothing, you may see people wearing gloves and masks to block the aerosol of pollens that could quickly invade the respiratory system. A popular over-the-counter item, swim goggles are designed to shield the eyes from pollens. They can also be inflated and release the pressure of small amounts of air that fill the goggles. Goggles, sometimes referred to as anti-fog and anti-bacterial supplies in the first aid kit, are a safety measure that can save the life of a person experiencing a severe allergic event. Following protocols and paying persistent attention to warning signs are the best ways to ensure continued protection for yourself and the safety of others.

When it comes to going outside with allergies, you want to take every preventative step possible to avoid potential allergic encounters. One way of doing so is by wearing allergy-friendly clothing. Choose shirts that are made with plastic-based fabrics and polar fleece. Stay away from wool, cashmere, silk, or cotton styles. Wool is a conductor of both heat and warm air. It will trap heat and make the body perspire and release moisture into the fabric. This warmth can trigger an allergic reaction if the fabric contains allergy-causing dust or if it is worn for a prolonged period of time. Wool has small fibers that irritate the skin and can cause severe allergic reactions with just one rub against the skin. The body's warmth and the air emitted during physical activity can also blow around mold and/or pollen. Touching your eyes with hands coated in pollen and/or mold will most assuredly result in an allergic response. The cold and heated air outdoors can cause your body's heart rate to constantly increase and decrease, making you feel cold while being active and warm when resting.

4. Choosing Allergy-Safe Locations

If there are no opportunities to determine the "purity" of the air based on research, it is assumed that frequent and significant rainfall contributes to cleansing the air of pollen. A parameter that also serves as an indicator of the highest health benefits of staying in tourist areas for people with allergies and other delicate health is the concentration of negative ions, which can also be determined by chemical air testing, but can be expected in sparsely urbanized as well as in land-use areas with a considerable amount of vegetation and water areas or in high mountains. Forest research scientists underline the importance of choosing which species of trees you want to see and where to go in a particular health condition. For example, hay fever is not advised to be in the presence of unfamiliar pollen varieties.

Having raised awareness of allergies and provided strategies for preparing allergy-friendly food and drinks, we can finally start our outdoor adventures. However, the choice of location is also important when planning it. Information about the level of pollen and pollen allergens has a limiting significance, which in practice means what really is in natural areas. In the context of looking for appropriate places without the risk of contact with allergens, especially anemophilic, for example, informed by friends who spent time outdoors in the area, as we also plan, the guidebooks and tourist brochures also have information on the preferred days and periods of stay in the area in terms of the pollen season.

4.1. Researching Pollen Levels and Air Quality

Pollen level and air quality measurements from different organizations provide information on the prevalence of pollen and air quality on most days but only provide details on the past few days. Since most weather forecasts provide information two to three weeks in advance, current and future pollen counts tend to go unobserved in local weather reports. Weather reports, including those from Accuweather and the Weather Channel, contain graphs representing the pollen levels for the past 5-7 days on that later share the pollen level in a written forecast. In addition to local weather and news station reports, there are more dedicated sources such as the Asthma and Allergy Foundation of America's (AAFA) national daily Allergy Capitals report. The most trustworthy predictions of upcoming wildland-fire smoky air conditions can be obtained from reliable city, county, state, federal, and private air quality management websites. These websites provide the most in-depth information regarding AQI, including monitoring data reports for pollutants and particular notices of air quality issues like smoky conditions from area wildfires.

When dealing with outdoor allergies, the first step to planning an outdoor trip is to research the pollen levels and air quality of the intended location(s) before deciding where to go. While pollen information is available through daily reports, air quality management (AQM) websites, and weather reports during spring, pollen-management websites as such do not provide a consolidated list of the places in the United States such as Hiking Project, All Trails, Adventure Projects, and other outdoor-based social media websites where pollen levels are minimal or non-existent based on the aridity and elevation of the outdoor location. Being able to identify places where a high number of species sufferers are less likely to encounter environmental allergens dramatically broadens the choices and opportunities for outdoor activities that individuals with severe allergies can participate in. Consequently, our objectives are to establish criteria and methods for analyzing AQM measures and reports from environmental allergen-suffering populations for identifying safe outdoor locations.

5. Managing Allergies During the Activity

When camping, cooking, or having a picnic, do not use scents or perfumes to avoid attracting stinging insects. If wearing a medical ID tag encourages you to be proactive or is a preferred strategy for you, feel free to use them. If you are out for a good run, swim, bike ride, hike, or strength training exercise, wear a cap to decrease pollen exposure and sunglasses to reduce drying of the ocular and nasal cavities. If you wear contact lenses and have allergies, consider using disposable lenses. Remove contact lenses as soon as possible after an allergen exposure to reduce the potential for prolonged ocular discomfort. Rinsing off after exposure to grass, near dandelions and allergenic plants, after a run, or during a hike can decrease allergen exposure for the remainder of the day. Engaging in behaviors to decrease allergen exposure and set the tone for the day can help you feel more comfortable.

It is important to assist children and adults in proactively managing allergic concerns when engaging in any new activities. The potency of most allergens rapidly diminishes within 20 minutes of the allergic encounter, but waiting a half-hour with an allergic reaction can be quite challenging for active youth or even active adults. Carry an oral antihistamine, an inhaler (if indicated), and an epinephrine autoinjector if prescribed. Before starting your activity, know how and when to access 911 and your local emergency response personnel and how to reach the local hospital.

Emergency contacts. Emergency contacts should be available to anyone with a known allergy. They can also help to dispel any doubt about the severity of an allergy if a reaction does occur. Include specialized contacts such as a personal allergist, nurse, or EMT; local medical centers or hospitals, as appropriate; and your emergency contact. Preparing this information can be a conversation starter with fellow campers and outdoor enthusiasts.

Emergency medications. Emergency medications should be available to anyone with a history of more severe or rapidly developing allergic reactions. Because even mild allergies can turn serious, a growing number of allergists recommend medications to a wider range of individuals. At any level of seriousness, addiction is almost impossible. The most important emergency medication to carry is an epinephrine autoinjector because it is effective at rapidly relieving the airway constriction and blood pressure loss that can occur during an allergic reaction. Two strengths are available, designed to deliver precise doses of epinephrine recommended for specific ages and weights of people.

Two things every person with allergies should carry are emergency medications and a list of emergency contacts. The medications should include an up-to-date epinephrine autoinjector, and the contacts should include the local emergency department. These two things help a person with allergies to feel proactive in case they have a reaction, but they also help to reinforce to others how truly important allergy assistance can be. For this reason, many experienced allergists recommend emergency medications even for mild allergies. Additional resources are available from the American College of Allergy, Asthma & Immunology, which also includes Spanish-language documentation. Materials are so useful that they have even been found on military calendars to prevent allergies at brush fires. Allergies are becoming more common, so actively discussing how to manage them during activities is an important conversation to have with campers and outdoor enthusiasts. Many will appreciate you for it, especially if they experience the fear of helplessness.

6. Post-Activity Care and Prevention

Finally, if an allergy has been discovered at any point, modify all previous activities to be achievable from a safe distance from the allergenic source. Asset mapping in the landscape can include an appreciation for the view from the car, which negates the need for further exposure to allergenic pollen or fungal spores. For those with comorbid hay fever or asthma, using air conditioning as a tool to avoid exposure is a useful trick, especially while taking remaining antihistamines during a ride home from a trip. For more information, please consult a board-certified allergist.

After a trip outdoors, it's imperative to shower and change clothes immediately. The former should be performed once allergenic exposure is complete or if clothing is soiled beyond what a mid-activity shake can handle. This prevents any contaminant from causing allergies to recur and reduces the occurrence of contact dermatitis. All clothing and equipment should be laundered as soon as possible post-activity to prevent any reactions following exposure once the gear is touched. Never leave dirty clothing or gear around the house where it can cause re-exposure. Some allergens can last for months without needing to be disturbed in order to reactivate, and this also prevents allergens from being reintroduced during the next use.

6.1. Showering and Changing Clothes Immediately

After physical activities are completed, follow your regular allergy management strategies which may include a daily antihistamine. Showering and washing your hair are essential to rinse outdoor allergens off your body. After you shower and dry off, consider putting on clean, outdoor-free clothing. When changing before bed, put your outdoor clothes in a closed hamper. "People put a lot of resources into what they do during sport or activity to help them decrease the likelihood of anaphylaxis, and what they do afterwards is super important, too, specifically in terms of prevention management – what are they doing to make sure that they wash off everything, not only off their body but also sleeves and cuffs, hats, shoes, all that stuff so they are not having constant re-exposures when they are doing outdoor activity," said Dr. Scott Hagan, Chief Investigator of the ALLERGIES study.

People with allergies are at a higher risk for anaphylaxis (severe allergic reactions) during and immediately following physical activities conducted outdoors. A significant way these individuals can stay safe and reduce the risk of an allergic event is to engage in vigilant preventative health practices. Physicians and other health professionals can work with patients and clients living with allergies to develop a comprehensive plan and educate them on the importance of taking care of themselves both during and following activity. Working in conjunction with a team of health professionals, people with allergies can enjoy successful, safe, and fun outdoor recreational endeavors and improve their health and overall well-being. These strategies are part of a second section of a study based on a survey published in 2021, "Exploring Allergies and Food Anaphylaxis: Enhancing Immune Resiliency in Active People (ALLERGIES IV) Survey."

Seasonal Allergy Management: Expert Advice for Outdoor Enthusiasts

1. Introduction to Seasonal Allergies

For many of us, pollen and the budding of gorgeous blossoms may cause havoc with our immune systems, prohibiting us from participating in recreational activities that we enjoy after being locked up all winter going through dry spell. With allergy season quickly approaching, we felt it was necessary to reach out to professionals on this subject in order to provide readers with various options to alleviate and even avoid discomfort. We questioned allergists to uncover the finest ways, medicines, or holistic cures for people who love to be outdoors but are hampered by their allergies. You can count on the fact that you're dealing with some of the greatest doctors and professionals in these fields, so let us help you unleash your spring self with these suggestions.

As we move into the spring equinox, the lovely seasonal perfection looks to be marred by a coating of charts and medications! As the climate begins to warm up, so too will one's nose! This is because springtime means different things to different people. Maybe wonderful weather, the return of outdoor sporting activities, and adventures are the most delightful aspects of this time of year. But aside from all the new activities available, the season is also distinguished for its high pollen levels. According to the American College of Allergy, Asthma, and Immunology, 23 million people suffer from seasonal allergies every year, and those numbers are climbing.

1.1. Understanding Seasonal Allergies

Seasonal allergies, also known as hay fever or allergic rhinitis, are most commonly caused by tree, grass, and weed pollen. The severity and duration of symptoms depend on the specific strain of pollen and the number of pollen grains in the air. Pollen count measures the amount of pollen present in the air. According to the Asthma and Allergy Foundation of America, pollen endemic regions in the United States had a majority of residents who said they had seasonal allergies. Grass pollen allergy, a common form of seasonal allergy, affects 10-30% of the people worldwide. The incidence of allergic rhinitis to trees and weeds is between 3 and 8% globally. Overall, as long as more pollen (i.e., allergens) are circulating through the environment, allergic rhinitis symptoms can last for several months.

Seasonal allergies are triggered by certain environmental factors, frequently airborne agents, that have been inhaled by the affected person. When the body's immune system declares certain allergens as abhorrent foreign bodies, typical allergic reactions often occur. Seasonal allergies, to put it another way, are caused by the very pollen grains that many outdoor adventurers and sports enthusiasts have been eagerly awaiting for the past several months. When pollen enters the nose, it can cause a cascade of allergy symptoms, such as a runny or stuffy nose, sneezing, a scratchy or sore throat, itchy or watery eyes, and wheezing in some situations. Even those who take care to avoid pollen and other airborne allergies will find it difficult when the pollen level peaks seasonally.

Seasonal allergies: What they are and how they affect sufferers

2. Common Triggers of Seasonal Allergies

When wildlife walk, inches behind them, they scatter about minuscule bits of dried-out excrement, hair, and feathers, also culminating in allergies. As such, feral cats and strays in city centers should be watched out for, especially when hitting the road. Goldenrod is very colloquially held as the main culprit of sneezy allergies, but in actuality, ragweed is typically the primary villain. It multiplies, releases, and surface-spores as the sky is dry and still. The plants open their tops during the summer months, when temperatures are moderate; strew their contents from August until October, when temp start to drop, and throughout, people run into issues.

A variety of environmental triggers may cause symptoms of allergies to arise, affecting the body in various ways, but mostly through the main system of sneezing, itching, and watery secretions. The most common trigger of seasonal allergies is pollen, a dust-like substance released into the air by trees, grasses, weeds, and during the summer and fall months. Mold spores, a fungus-induced alternative to pollen, is a mushroom-like substance that forms in outdoor or indoor environments that are wet or humid. Mold counts typically rise in response to rain or moisture, and in dry climates or high-altitude areas with low relative indoor humidity, such as the South and Midwest, mold counts are generally lower. Additionally, climate plays a role in high mold counts, with the existence of humidity frequently inflating values in warmer regions. Other common outdoor allergen triggers include pet dander, tiny flakes from an animal's skin, in addition to insect stings, which disturb the immune system.

2.1. Pollen

Avoid activity in a windstorm or on warmer and drier mornings. Maintain low exertion levels during spring, typically 5:30 am to 10:30 am, when pollen counts are highest. Be mindful of pollen counts during the summer months. Rainstorms can reduce the pollen count on the day of the rain, but within a few hours of the rain stopping, the pollen count can increase rapidly. Try not to start outdoor activities within a few hours of the rain stopping. For more information, it's advised to check or download the pollen counts for locations through websites such as NationalAllergy.com.

Tips and Tactics

Allergies to pollen affect many Americans and are a trigger for symptoms year-round. Tree pollen is an early spring allergy culprit, while grass pollen can peak in May through June. Weeds may produce allergic reactions starting in late spring and lasting into early fall. The height of the growing season typically corresponds to the most plant growth and pollen activity. During this time, millions of small, almost invisible protein particles are released into the air by plants. Most pollen pieces are 10-20 microns large, which are large enough to make the air particles hazy or slightly tinted in color at times. They are small enough, however, to be blown into the deepest lung passages or even into the bloodstream. Pollen counts can surge during the light to moderate wind speeds found in the mountains. An average day in the mountains, usually slightly breezy, will almost always kick up the pollen count in the local air. Many outdoor enthusiasts feel the effects of seasonal allergies.

In-Depth

Pollen is produced by plants to spread seeds. This facilitator of new plant growth is a common cause of seasonal allergies.

The One Thing

2.2. Mold Spores

First off, get a handle on when the season starts. While molds are present year-round, some types release spores in the warmer months and thrive in the humid summer air. Mold counts are especially high during foggy, high-humidity days when wind currents keep the moisture-laden air from leaving the area. If mold season is making the beginning of your week rough, consider your options for relieving outdoor allergies after the jump.

For patients with mold allergies:

In many cases, avoiding mold is very similar to avoiding pollen. However, keeping an eye on the mold count in addition to the pollen count may give those allergic to mold some warning to stay indoors.

- Moldy hay (and other decaying plant material) - Dumps, cellars, basements - Anywhere with poor ventilation - Other areas with poor ventilation - Rain gutters - Compost piles - Rotten wood, especially damp fence boards and wood used for buildings - Leaf litters - Wheat fields - Damp musty areas of barns and houses - Places with high humidity and poor air circulation

Some of the common mold allergy triggers include:

It's no secret that mold is a major outdoor allergen. It's a year-round problem for those with indoor allergies and a major issue in the outdoor environment for part of the year. Mold allergy symptoms are often identical to those caused by pollen, and it is likely that many patients who believe they are allergic to pollen are also reacting to mold.

2.3. Pet Dander

Should this approach ultimately fail to provide relief for an individual with seasonal allergies, the best option will be to discuss the issue with an allergist, Pien said. "If someone is being sidelined because they are unable to tolerate the treatment or they are not having an effect from the treatment, that would be a very good person to discuss this with," he said. "If someone is that severely affected by their allergies, they really owe it to themselves to see an allergist and have that approach completely evaluated." People who are already using nearly all the available medications and staying indoors may want to consider this option as well.

While some outdoor enthusiasts are able to find some relief by limiting their activity to areas with fewer trees, some animals that produce pet dander, a common seasonal allergy trigger, such as cats, will be active in any location. Pet dander is often encountered in public gathering spaces and is present in homes and other buildings, so those allergic to pet dander may find it particularly challenging to avoid exposure. To minimize the impact of pet dander (and other potential allergen) exposure, always take preventive medication before spending time outdoors. For those who use preventive treatment, it may also be useful to bring along oral or nasal medication that can be taken during outdoor activities if allergies flare up, DeMera added. There are a growing number of medications (both over-the-counter and by prescription) available to relieve allergy symptoms. Talk to an allergist about your options.

3. Preparing for Outdoor Activities

Within 24 hours of the outing, rivals may seem to surprise you by increasing their output against you (which, statistically speaking, means there's a good chance this is prime time for tree pollen levels). They recommend checking the day's Pollen Index Score (PIS) at the American Academy of Allergy, Asthma & Immunology website. On days when the PIS for tree pollen is high: Take your medications. Remember, nasal antihistamines and allergen-eye drops can help you avoid eye- and hand-rubbing flare-ups later in the day. Applying medicated nasal spray about 8-12 hours before your planned outing may help protect you from the effects of particulate rehab for at least part of the day. Wearing sunglasses appear to help keep allergens farther from your eyes.

Planning outdoor activities can exacerbate anxiety when it's not just the weather that can add plot twists to a planned outdoor excursion. However, you can decrease the "yikes" factor by taking the proper precautions and preparing yourself in advance. We've asked the pros at American Academy of Allergy, Asthma & Immunology (AAAAI) for their advice. Here is some guidance for people with seasonal (aka pollen) allergies and who also are avid outdoor enthusiasts and want to be outdoors to hike a trail, bike a path, ride a bike on a trail, or run a race.

3.1. Check Pollen Counts

To help predict what outdoor enthusiasts might be going through, take a look at websites such as [website], which provides a 5-day allergy forecast and a 10-day pollen forecast, with counts for four different types of pollen: tree, grass, weed, and mold. These counts are scaled from 0 to 12; a count of 9-12 is considered high, and a count of 0-2 is considered low. Another good website is [website], which also predicts pollen levels in 5-day increments and features tracked pollen types, providing information on different tree species.

Here are some of the common symptoms that are often attributed to seasonal allergies: nasal congestion, runny nose, sneezing, postnasal drainage, itchy nose, itchy throat, itchy ears, itchy eyes, red eyes, watery eyes, cough, sore throat, hoarse voice, and the absence of a fever. It is virtually impossible to avoid pollen when you are outside, but working to minimize exposure can make participation in outdoor activities much more enjoyable.

Before heading out on any outdoor adventure, check the pollen count in the area you plan to visit. High pollen counts can trigger outdoor allergy symptoms. At the very least, focusing on the pollen count can help you mentally prepare for what's to come. High counts can also indicate that your symptoms may be more severe. Pro tip: because new pollen is released in the early morning, pollen counts are low late in the afternoon.

3.1 Check pollen counts.

Expert advice for outdoor enthusiasts with seasonal allergies: A collection of practical tips.

3.2. Choose the Right Time of Day

Knowing the weather is a good start when trying to plan the best activity times. Cities like even have detailed tallies of what allergens are plaguing your area. But keeping track of the hourly pollination reports, typically given from 5 a.m. to 5 p.m. solid, will give you the complete picture. Ragweed is known for sending pollen soaring during your work day, while tree pollination fades out by the evening. If you want to take a break and walk away from your computer, standard allergies were good, but avoid the mid-day rambles. Always do gardening or mowing in the evening. When pollen is first released, it rises into the air forming layers or pools of pollens. In the early hours of the day, these layers mix with cooler air which can block the pollen release. By around 7:30 am-8:30 am the sun has warmed the ground sufficiently to break up pool and into convected columns of air can carry the pollen aloft.

Not all times of day are created equal in terms of pollen dispersal and concentration in the air. Some of the best times of day to engage in outdoor activities if you suffer from allergies are the times after a storm. Pollen tends to settle due to the wet air and lower temperatures associated with storms. Pollen travels the least on cold days, so activities during or immediately following storms are at a time when there may be less pollen in the air. Windy and warm days have the highest pollen production. This can be mid-to-late morning because it takes a little more warmth to start the pollination process. It's also good in the evening when it's cooling off. The days that are really sunny and bright are the best days for temperature contrast. The pollen behaves in different ways depending on the type of particle that is being emitted.

4. Managing Allergy Symptoms

Here are several of the best over-the-counter and alternative remedies to consider for those with minor to more severe seasonal allergies: over-the-counter antihistamines and decongestants; oral and nasal antihistamines for fast relief; steroidal nose sprays; leukotriene inhibitors. However, if the idea of taking medications concerns you, allergy experts and outdoor recreation professionals have other suggestions. "Allergy season can be unbearable for an outdoor enthusiast, so it's important to arm yourself with the best remedies," confirms Nick of BikingGuides.com. Wildlife Advisor offers 7 natural remedies that are sure to lower the degree of those bothersome seasonal allergies. Topping her list is "quercetin. It's a compound that works well at reducing inflammation," says Joe Hannagan, PhD.

According to Dr. Knox, the two classes of over-the-counter seasonal allergy medications that might help you are antihistamines and decongestants. Antihistamines work by blocking histamines, which cause inflammation and itching; decongestants work by constricting the blood vessels in the nose to help open up the passages. These can be used at the same time. However, he also says that often, over-the-counter treatments won't manage more severe allergy symptoms. If you find yourself feeling miserable or struggling with a dangerous allergy, experts urge you to seek care from a board-certified allergist who can evaluate symptoms and develop a comprehensive treatment plan, including a solution involving over-the-counter or prescription medication, based on personalized testing.

4.1. Over-the-Counter Medications

Seasonal allergy symptoms are reflections of the immune system's response to foreign particles entering and aggravating the nasal mucosal tissue. Histamine is a mediator that plays a major role in allergy symptoms, creating an environment favorable for sneezing, itching, rhinorrhea, and nasal congestion. Antihistamines, or H1 antagonists, are medications that alter the action of histamine on H1 receptors, thereby preventing the release of histamine and symptom onset or relapse. Antihistamines are frequently taken as a preventive measure for all seasonal allergy sufferers, but can also be used for treatment of acute symptoms. Both the 1st-generation and 2nd-generation antihistamines have been submitted as monograph ingredients for relief of seasonal allergic rhinitis. Fexofenadine is also approved as an OTC medication for the relief of hives and skin itching due to hives. Antihistamines are well tolerated at suggested doses and have few side effects. The 1st-generation antihistamines could have sedative or drowsiness side effects in users.

A variety of over-the-counter medications and complementary therapies are available to help manage symptoms of seasonal allergies. We discuss a number of treatment prevention, treatment, and monitoring measures for individuals with seasonal allergies; however, certain measures are suitable for a general sports medicine practice. Topical and oral decongestants, oral antihistamines, and mast cell stabilizers are available over the counter for allergic rhinitis. The effectiveness of these medications may not be as strong as prescription counterparts, but they are not without merit, particularly as short-term symptom relief. Moreover, they may be most appealing to very physically active individuals who desire immediate relief with minimal potential for adverse events that could impede their exercise or physical activity. Some might be particularly well tolerated, with less potential for secondary drowsiness, congestion, or 'rebound' effects. Knowledge and use of these products, indication, adverse effects, and appropriate usage could better assist individuals seeking nonpharmacologic and nonprescription recommendations.

4.2. Prescription Medications

It is not always true that if you take twice the dose of an OTC medication it will be as effective as the prescription strength. There are safe upper limits for each OTC medication and any OTC medications when combined with prescription medications. Therefore, the best way to find the right approach is to work with your healthcare provider to ensure you are getting the optimal dosing and regimen to achieve relief for your symptoms while minimizing the risk of side effects.

The difference between the OTC versions and prescription medications is their dosage and their route of administration. Nasal sprays that contain antihistamines or corticosteroids are also available and can be beneficial in controlling nasal symptoms. If you have been using over-the-counter medications at the appropriate doses and feel you are not getting relief, speak with your medical provider about the possibility of trying a short course of prescription medications or receiving prescription treatments that can help with unmanaged symptoms, especially when the medications interfere with your ability to do certain activities.

- Oral antihistamines: levocetirizine, fexofenadine - Nasal antihistamine: azelastine - Nasal steroids: many choices including fluticasone and triamcinolone

While over-the-counter (OTC) antihistamines are safe and effective for many people, about 20% of individuals with seasonal allergies do not get the relief they need from OTC treatments. Prescription medications, which are available as over-the-counter medications at higher doses, have been found to be more effective in managing seasonal allergy symptoms. Antihistamines are also available in eye drops that provide a more direct route of administration and may be particularly useful for individuals in whom eye symptoms are prominent.

4.3. Natural Remedies

There are hundreds of complementary therapy approaches for reacting to environmental problems, ranging from elements of the Traditional Chinese Medicine (TCM) and Ayurvedic medicine paradigms to the Homeopathic, to Naturopathic, Herbal, Western physiological and energetic, to physical therapies and mind-body therapies. An overview of every flavor or approach like TCM, Naturopathic or Homeopathic remedies would be a book unto itself, so we focus here on the natural remedies (other than pharmaceutical antihistamines, decongestants and corticosteroid nasal sprays or leukotriene antagonists) that have had some level of investigation of allergenic, and sometimes asthmatic, mechanisms and/or symptoms such as inflammation.

The previous sections cover some of the pharmaceutical and immunological interventions and strategies for outdoor activity management that can help to minimize the impact of worker allergies or asthma symptoms. However, a more subset group in the allergy population and superset needs and preferences in the general population are interested in natural therapies as alternatives for managing their symptoms. They ask for 'natural' remedies and are generous with their spending on natural remedies, as well as other non-pharmaceutical interventions. However, gold standard evidence for many natural remedies is not robust. While initially positive, many meta-analyses reveal concerns of bias in the reporting of positive study results, potentially confounded results due to the lack of a standard for 'placebo' in natural therapy research. They also often show 'relationships' without confirmed 'cause and effect' as the protective immunity associated with eating one apple/day is unlikely to be created by the ellagic acid content of the fruit, because if this were so, for heart health, one would only ever need to eat one bowl of porridge! Natural remedies are not without risks. Everything that you consume to 'act to benefit' you may also have the potential of an unwanted effect and the potential to interact with prescribed medicines.

5. Allergy Prevention Tips

These hints can improve the quality of life for those who suffer from seasonal allergies and are written with an active, preventionist mindset that may appeal to those who frequently spend time outdoors. Formatted into a list, the information feels less dense and more digestible, leading people to take these tips more seriously. Taking allergy medication a couple of hours before the hike, however, promises relief that takes effect longer before the actual hike while not making a time-consuming snack stop on the day-of.

- Monitor pollen counts and avoid outdoor activities on high pollen count days. - If you are outdoors during high pollen count days, try to limit outdoor activities to early morning or after a good rain and avoid peak pollen shed times (10 a.m. - 4 p.m.). - Shower and shampoo after outdoor activities to remove pollen from skin and hair; rinse eyes with saline eye drops to remove pollen. - Change outdoor clothing and wash it immediately when returning indoors. - Avoid hanging linens and clothes outside to dry: pollen may stick to these items. - Plan outdoor activities that require physical exertion on low pollen count days because pollen exposure increases at higher speeds during activities such as biking, running, and playing basketball. - Short-acting over-the-counter antihistamines and decongestants can be used to decrease allergy symptoms. Be aware that antihistamines can cause drowsiness. Non-drowsy antihistamines can be purchased containing fexofenadine (Allegra), loratadine (Claritin, Alavert), or cetirizine (Zyrtec). Medications should be taken 1-2 hours prior to outdoor activities for the best effect.

Avoidance is the single most effective method for managing allergies. This section provides a series of practical tips for preventing seasonal allergies in outdoor settings.

5.1. Wear Protective Clothing

Consider inquired advice for enacting strategies to reduce contact between allergens, clothing, skin, or hair/skin. Research outdoor clothing and gear that reduces potential allergenic contact, such as sunglasses, eye shield, goggle, hat, headband, face mask, and neck/backpacks. Specialized outdoor catalogs or website resources can provide products for use during recreational outdoor activities such as gardening, hiking, camping, sporting events, or commercial or professional activities. Hats should have solid or mesh fabric to cover the scalp. Avoid sun hats designed to protect only from the sun. Wear a non-woven disposable mask or washable mask in a cotton wallet or front pocket. Facemask pocket should be fabric not less than 2-3 microns or 100% cotton. Wearing such eczema-friendly protectants should reduce the amount and duration of pollen contact on the face and neck. Protectants that are reusable or washable are considered to be more environmentally and economically friendly. The top band along the forehead protects the face as well if the mask slips or is removed.

During the pollen season, wear clothes that are specially designed to be worn to prevent pollen from coming into contact with your skin. This can protect the region of skin directly exposed to pollen from the elements. For instance, the mask or gator shields your mouth and nose against inhalation of allergens, while wearing a cap or sunhat can help safeguard the hair and scalp against allergenic pollen particles. Select clothes that are made of tightly woven material, based on appropriate criteria such as the size of the pores and the quantity or weight of the fabrics, to avoid the penetration of pollen to the skin.

Subsection 5.1. Wear Protective Clothing

5.2. Shower After Outdoor Activities

If you are allergic to pollen, dust mite, and dander (fleas) or you are not sure what you are allergic to, it is beneficial to shower your hair with soap and water, and gently scrub into the scalp to remove as much dander as possible. The face should also be thoroughly washed to remove pollen and dust before gently drying yourself with a clean towel and putting on clean clothes. If you leave these allergens on your skin or in your hair and on your clothing, you can continue to experience itchy, allergic reactions. If you cannot shower after outdoor activities, at a minimum, using baby wipes to wipe down your skin and face can also be beneficial for itchy, allergic reactions. To recall, sections 5.1 and 5.2 suggest avoiding specific circumstances to prevent allergic reactions as an expert's strategy for the downwind outdoor enthusiast. It has further been suggested that leaving what is likely to make one reactive is a precaution for those with allergies.

While getting pollen on your skin, hair, and clothing is unavoidable if you are enjoying outdoor activities, you can prevent seasonal allergies by managing your hygiene post-activity. Dermatologists suggest changing clothes and showering as soon as possible to prevent skin reactions, and this advice can also help prevent allergic reactions. Promptly removing your shoes and changing clothes from long hikes, runs, and bike rides will prevent pollen from being spread throughout your living space. This also helps reduce repeated contact with pollen, which can prevent prolonged allergic symptoms. Showering promptly will remove most of the pollen on your skin and hair, helping to prevent it from soaking into clothes or keeping you awake with itchy night. During the night time, when the body repairs itself, the histamine reaction to pollen can be very strong for those who are allergic.

6. Consulting with a Physician

Long-term medications can help manage severe allergy symptoms, but long-term use of some medications may exceed drug tolerance or have some side effects. The best answer to this question depends on many different factors, both personal and specific symptoms, to the patient themselves. A physician is a patient in the future who can help them in patient care decisions.

If the symptoms of seasonal allergies interfere with your life, do not hesitate to consult with a professional because it can last a long time. Pharmaceutical therapies may reduce the severity of allergy entered after symptoms appear, but the use of immunotherapy is a preventive option so that the symptoms do not worsen in the first place.

Consult with a professional doctor or physician. With the help of the doctor, trying to manage the impact of seasonal allergies can provide medical advice for the following personalized needs. Information about the symptoms can be very helpful in assessing the potential and disease-specific medications or therapy regimens that can be effective for indoors and outdoors.

Certainly. Details provided in section 6 are discussed below.

6.1. When to Seek Medical Advice

- Sudden, severe shortness of breath. - Severe wheezing and coughing. - A blue tinge to the skin or lips (cyanosis). - Tightness in the chest that does not get better with medication. - These signs are particularly ominous in someone who has never previously had asthma. If they occur, get emergency help immediately. In the setting of known asthma, this symptom complex may still require an ambulance transport to an emergency room for further clinical evaluation. Although asthma is a serious and potentially life-threatening disease when poorly treated or left unaddressed, it is more often associated with quality treatment than with fatal outcomes. With appropriate asthma management, most patients who experience the above symptoms still do quite well in the long term. However, the cornerstone of any preventative treatment is early recognition of warning symptoms.

- You are regularly missing work, school, or events because of your allergies. - Over-the-counter treatments are no longer providing you with relief. - You are having increasing symptoms in spite of conservative allergy avoidance techniques. - Also, some symptoms you may be experiencing can signal the start of an asthma attack, especially in the case of pollen allergies triggering asthma, and this should prompt you to seek emergency help. Some possible triggers of serious asthma attacks might include the sudden and unexpected onset of life-threatening symptoms such as:

In general, you should seek medical advice if your allergy symptoms are significantly affecting your quality of life. Some signs that it is time to see a doctor include but are not limited to: